Treat Infection Naturally

By
Lynne D M Noble

Copyright 2018 Lynne D M Noble

Independently published

Contents

Dedication

To Michael

Preface

Before antibiotics were discovered, people had to think up other ways of combatting diseases which could cause disfigurement or be ultimately fatal, if not treated. Those with tuberculosis were treated with fresh air. That is, their wheeled wicker beds were placed outside in the sunshine. This rest therapy worked because there was less stress on the immune system. The sunshine provided vitamin D, which as we shall see is important in combatting infection. Finally, the physical position of the individual also deprived the tuberculosis organism of oxygen. The mycobacterium organism depends on oxygen for survival and the lying down position deprives the bacterium of it.

Of course, the recuperation periods in the sanatorium were long. Not everyone survived but this is no less true, nowadays. It may be less true in the future as   antibiotic resistance continues to eat into the few drugs that we have left and we have forgotten the old ways of combatting disease.

We live in fast society where no one has time to lie out on a wicker bed to recuperate – or indeed any bed. We expect to be dished out antibiotics so that we can go back to work or take up our life more or less immediately. We even demand antibiotics when we have infections which antibiotics don't work on such as viruses or fungal diseases. The result of all this, is that a bacterium has already been found which is resistant to any antibiotic.

Bacteria are clever organisms. They have defence systems which work against some antibiotics but, generally, not all of them. However, they can pass on their defence systems onto other bacteria who don't have the arsenal of weapons that they have. Eventually, as different bacteria pass on their own specific weapons to others, the bacteria will be collecting a full arsenal of weapons. At this point antibiotics will be totally useless against this new superbug.

The first antibiotic was discovered in 1928 by Alexander Fleming. In 1945 Fleming received the

Nobel prize for medicine. He was already warning about antibiotic resistance at this point – just 17 years after his discovery.

Of course scientists are always looking for new antibiotics but, regardless of this, global resistance will be a reality one day. The good news is there many natural anti-microbials around us which are able to treat many infective agents and we have the best defences, in the form of our immune system, which is an amazing creation. We can even produce our own anti-microbials from foods that we eat.

Once you understand this, you can take control back from the over reliance you have on prescribed medication Further, you can harness the amazing power of our immune system and understand why many common foods and substances have the power against disease that they do have.

This book will look at many common antimicrobials which are readily available as well as the common conditions that they address. Further, we will take a look at the immune system and learn the difference between innate and adaptive immunity and how to keep both in tip top condition. When the immune system is running at optimum levels then many infections are destroyed before you are even aware of any symptoms.

The Immune System

The purpose of the immune system is to prevent infection such as bacteria, viruses and fungi out of the body. If any do invade the body, then the immune system will attempt to seek and destroy them.

The immune system has two parts. The

- **Innate immune system** which are the barriers that the body has such as the
  a. Cough reflex
  b. Skin
  c. Enzymes in tears
  d. Skin oils
  e. Stomach acid
  f. Mucus which traps bacteria and small particles

and

- **The acquired immune system** which consists of white blood cells (lymphocytes) and antibodies.

The innate immune system is a non-specific defence mechanism that starts defending the body within hours of an invader appearing in the body. Undamaged skin is an excellent barrier for keeping infection out but if it becomes damaged, or dry, then germs can penetrate. It is clear then that if an injury occurs or the skin is dry and scaly - as can happen in skin conditions like psoriasis and eczema – then the risk of infection is greatly increased.

Mucus in the respiratory tract helps trap germs and the cough reflex helps them be coughed back up the respiratory tract where they are often swallowed.

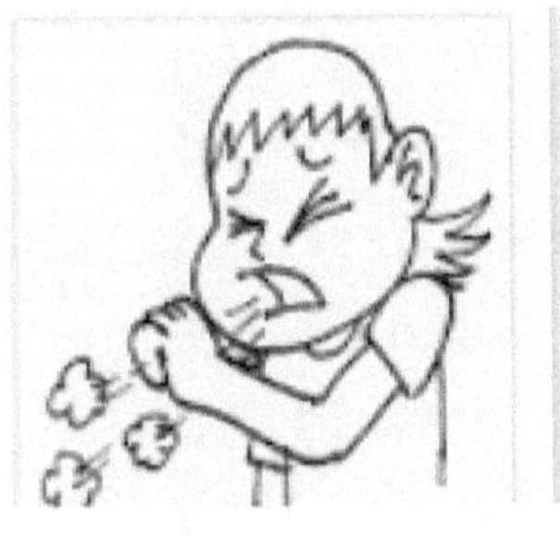

In the stomach, the acid – which has a pH of 2 – destroys anything it comes

1

---

1 https://slideplayer.com/slide/4191151/

into contact with. Anybody who has had heartburn will know how strong stomach acid is.

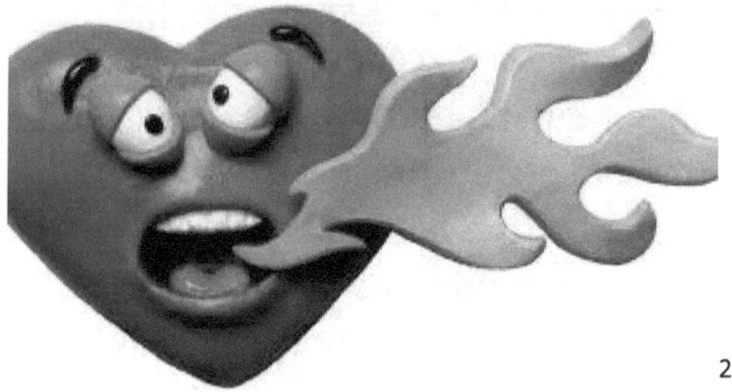

2

Problems occur when people take antacids and the pH is less acidic. This can allow for all sorts of bugs to flourish which will make us ill.

Conditions such as heartburn and indigestion increase with age. The muscle at the bottom of the food pipe (oesophagus) becomes laxer and allows the acid to escape. The problem is the sphincter muscle but people take antacids to cope with the symptoms. In doing so, they compromise one of their defences.

---

2 http://asianworldnews.co.uk/health/reduce-acid-reflux-or-heartburn-by-strengthening-the-les-valve/

Whereas the innate immune system generally takes up a defensive position the adaptive or acquired immune system is the armed forces of the immune system.

If any infective agent breaches the innate defences then white cells called Helper T cells receive signals from the white blood cells of the innate system, such as phagocytes and relay them to the warriors of the adaptive defences. These are the B cells and cytoxic T cells.

The B cells bind to germs and this labels them as needing to be destroyed.

There is a second class of B cells called memory cells. They remember invading germs which have been destroyed. If such a germ tries to invade again in the future then the B cell, having had prior experience of it, react much more quickly to the invader.

The cytoxic T cells can detect viruses which hide inside the host cell. Our cells present bits of molecules on the surface of their cells. If they are foreign, then the cytoxic T cells send signals to the infected cell instructing them to commit suicide. While this kills off the host cell, it also kills off the virus.

The adaptive immune system reacts to specific germs whereas the innate immune system is more general in response.

The body makes its own antibodies. These are acquired either actively or passively.

Examples of passively acquired antibodies are the IgG which is passed from the maternal placenta to the unborn child. IgG and IgA are also passed onto the new born in colostrum and mother's milk when feeding the new born.

Active immunity occurs when people make their own antibodies in response to infection or vaccination.

Each white blood cell can only recognise one particular molecular shape on top of a germ. Some can recognise shapes for bacteria which cause strep throats and others can only recognise shapes for staphylococci which tend to be the infecting agent for skin infections such as boils. When they recognise their own shape they become activated. They attach to antigens and this marks them for destruction by other cells such as phagocytes which surround them and engulf them.

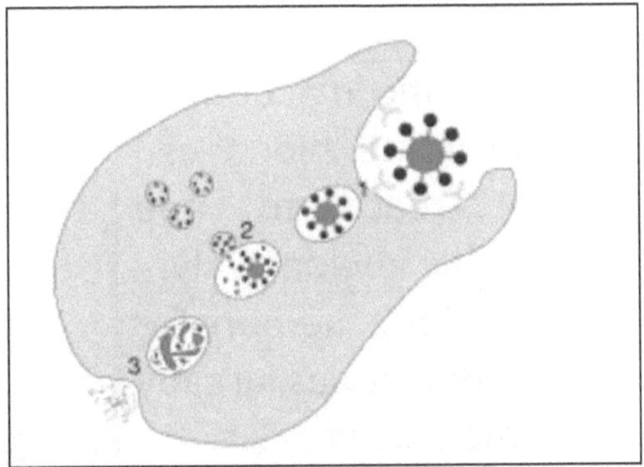

Phagocyte engulfing an antigen[3]

The phagocyte produces hydrogen peroxide which also helps to kill the invader. Honey also contains hydrogen peroxide which is why it is used on dressings for infected wounds.

---

[3] https://sciencing.com/two-types-phagocytes-8544033.html

<u>Table showing some of the main differences in the innate immune system and the adaptive/acquired immune system.</u>

Innate immune system	Adaptive immune system
Responds quickly to invaders	Is slower to respond
Has a non-selective action	Is specific in action. Eg one white blood cell will react to one specific invader only
Does not make memory cells	Has a long memory for invaders it has already come across.
Composed of a number of defensive reflex actions and substances eg the cough reflex or mucus which is used to trap invaders	Composed of white blood cells and antibodies

Side Effects of Antibiotics

There is no doubt that the discovery of antibiotics has helped save many lives but they also have a great many side effects which can, in some cases, prove life-threatening. Some antibiotics create more negative side effects than others. Some of these side effects can interfere with the patient's ability to tolerate and finish the course of medication.

Common side effects of antibiotics include:

- Upset stomach
- Diarrhoea
- Rashes
- Fungal infections like thrush

Sometimes there are more severe allergic reactions which can result in difficulty breathing and facial swelling or there can be severe bloody diarrhoea.

Some years ago I was prescribed clarithromycin for a chest infection. I hadn't been prescribed this antibiotic before but, as I had never had problems with antibiotics before, it never entered my head that I would this time.

I was in our village at the time. I stopped off for a drink on the way home and took the capsule then carried on my way home. I remember feeling a little lightheaded and a little unsteady but, of course, I wasn't well and I'd had quite a busy day.

The rest of the day passed uneventfully until I took the second dose at about 7.30pm. Shortly after I had taken it I felt distinctly unwell. A visitor had arrived and I recall just wanting them to go because I thought I was going to pass out. They left and I managed to stagger to the settee. I was very tachycardic and I thought I was going to pass out again. I couldn't have got up off the settee but I did manage to telephone the ambulance service.

They confirmed that I was tachycardic and I was taken to the crash room at the local hospital where I continued to have irregular bouts of tachycardia for a couple of hours before I was allowed to go home. I will never take clarithromycin again and, in fact, was informed by the medical team that I should not in the future.

One of the unwanted side effects of antibiotics which tends not to reach the leaflets enclosed with the medication is that can produce significant weight gain.

Gut bacteria have numerous functions in your body and can play a role in obesity. Studies have shown that exposure to antibiotics in early life may have long term consequences for a child's metabolism.

Mice given antibiotics for the first four weeks of life grew up to be 25% heavier. They also had 60% more body fat than the controls.

Earlier research also showed that mice fed antibiotics – in doses similar to those given to children for throat or ear infections had significant increases in body fat despite their diets remaining unchanged.

There is an association between the composition of the intestinal microbiota and obesity. This has been demonstrated by studies showing differences in microbiota composition between obese and lean humans.

Obesity is associated with an increase of the phylum Firmucutes and a decrease in Bacteroidetes which are partly attributable to diet.

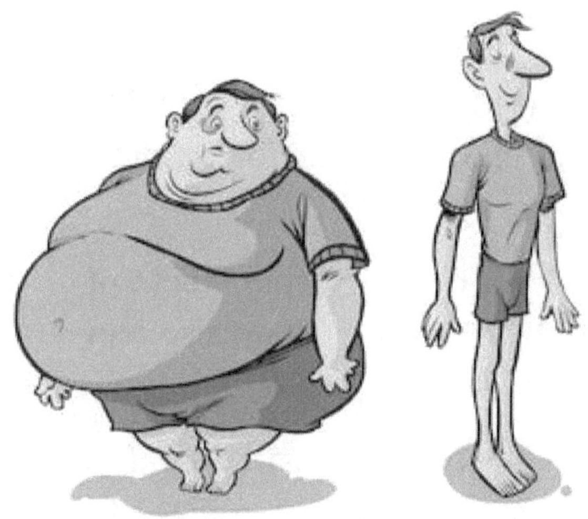

Left: microbiota of increased Firmucute. Right: microbiota of increased Bacteroidetes

When a low energy diet is taken then there is a shift in gut microbiota with a decrease in

Firmucutes similar in composition to that of a lean person.

Since the judicious use of antibiotics is now of paramount importance and further, that they do not work on many infectious agents such as viruses, then we need to look further at some alternative remedies for common ailments. Further, we also need to look at how we can harness our own defences.

Vitamin D – immune system regulator

Vitamin D is one of the unsung heroes of the vitamin world. When people think about vitamin D – if they do at all - they think of it in association with healthy bones. Most people do not realise that vitamin D makes its own antimicrobial called cathelicidin. Further, as the majority of the world are vitamin D deficient, this suggests that the majority of the world aren't harnessing the power within their own immune systems.

An antimicrobial is an agent that kills microorganisms or stops their growth. Cathelicidins are small antimicrobial peptides. They are part of our innate immune system and show a broad spectrum of antimicrobial activity against

- Bacteria
- Enveloped viruses
- Fungi

As well as exerting direct antimicrobial effects such as punching holes in the cell membranes of invaders, the cathelicidins can also trigger specific defence responses in the host.

Vitamin D upregulates the production of cathelicidins and is found to exert an effect in many organs and systems of the body. This is not surprising since vitamin D receptors can be found throughout the body.

Cathelicidins have been found in the:

- Stomach
- Trachea
- Skin
- Muscle
- Heart
- Kidney
- Lung
- Brain
- Intestine

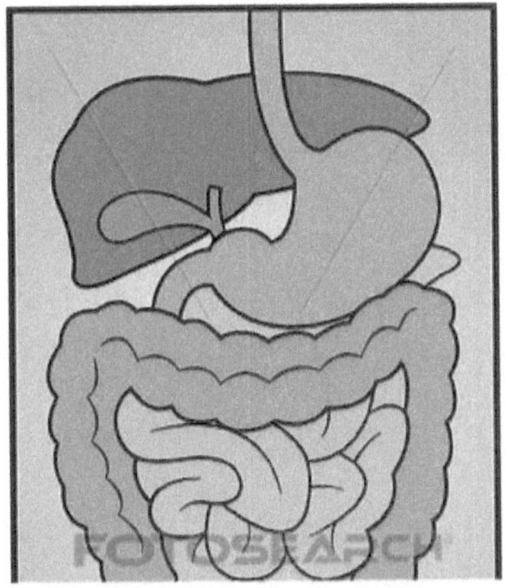

Cathelicidins have been found in the digestive system.

Human cathelicidin acts in the promotion of wound healing and can modulate the adaptive immune system.

Higher plasma levels of human cathelicidin antimicrobial protein, which are upregulated by vitamin D, appear to significantly reduce the risk of death from infection in dialysis patients. Studies show that patients with a high level of this protein were 3.7 times more likely to survive kidney dialysis for a year without a fatal infection.   This shows how powerful this natural antimicrobial is.

As people get older they are less likely to be able to absorb vitamin D through their skin. Older people and those with inflammatory bowel disease have greater difficulty absorbing any nutrient from food. Further, it is extremely difficult, if not impossible, to obtain sufficient vitamin D from the diet.

The best sources of vitamin D are oily fish, fortified cereals and eggs. However, you would need to eat 80 eggs daily to obtain sufficient vitamin D for the day.   The recommended daily amount is 1000-4000 IU's.

Supplements are advised for

- The elderly
- Those who are housebound
- Those who work indoors
- Those with black skin
- Those with inflammatory bowel disease or other conditions where the ability to absorb nutrients is compromised.

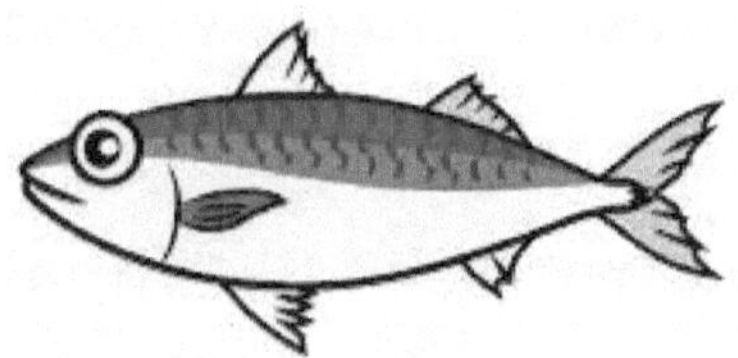

Oily fish such as mackerel, salmon and fresh tuna contain good amounts of vitamin D.

Medium Chain Fatty Acids

Medium chain fatty acids (MCFA's) are chains of fatty acids which are 6-12 chains long. Due to their length they have special properties. They can be used directly by the liver as a source of energy or they can be changed into ketones. Ketones are substances which the liver produces when it breaks down large amounts of fat for energy.

 Ketones can cross the blood brain barrier and be used as fuel instead of glucose which the brain normally uses.

MCFA's are less likely to be turned into fat as they can so easily be turned into energy for immediate use.

Just from this perspective they can be an immediate source of energy when you are ill.

The main sources of MCFA's can be seen in the table below.

Type of MCFA	Source of MCFA's
C6 – caproic acid(hexanoic acid)	butter
C8 – caprylic acid (octanoic acid)	Coconut oil, palm kernel oil, goat cheese, butter
C10 – capric acid – (decanoic acid)	Coconut oil, palm kernel oil
C12 – Lauric acid – (dodecanoic acid)	Coconut oil

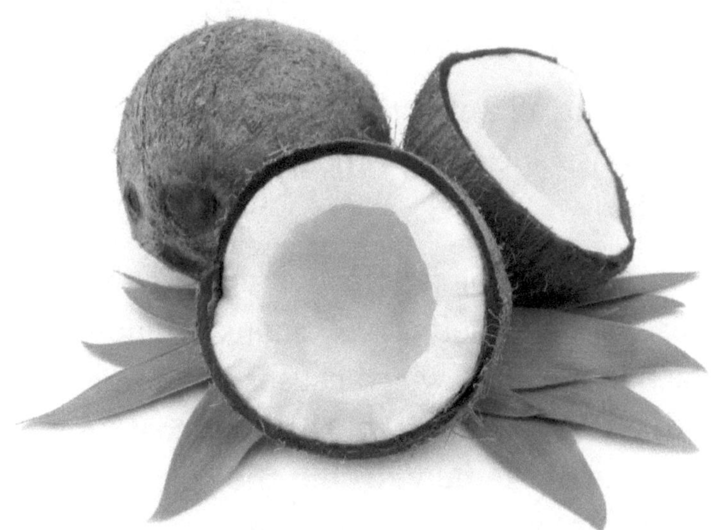

Coconut oil has antibacterial, antifungal, antiviral and antiprotozoal actions in the body. Its unique fatty acids Breast milk contains MCFA's. It helps protect the baby when its own immune system is hardly developed.

Studies have shown that MCFA's are effective against viruses causing measles, influenza, pneumonia, throat infections, herpes and AIDS. MCFA'S also are effective against bacteria causing pneumonia, throat infections, stomach infections, sinusitis, rheumatic fever, urinary tract infections, meningitis and dental cavities.

MCFA's are also effective against many fungal infections including those which cause thrush.

While coconut oil is effective against the flu virus, it is not effective against rhinovirus which is the virus which causes the common cold. The MCFA's act on the lipid coating or envelope of the flu virus but the cold virus is not enveloped in a lipid coating.

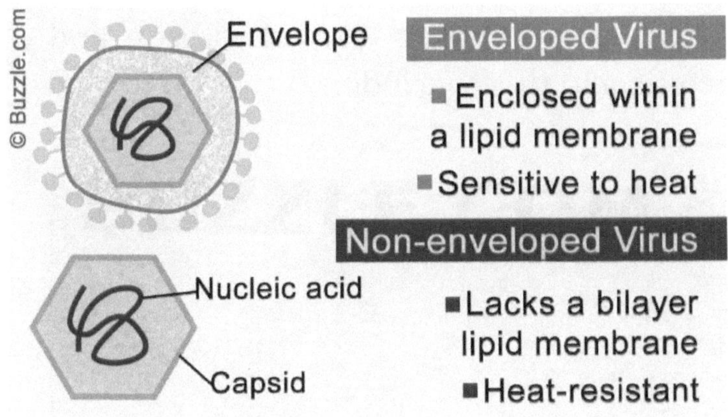

However, we do not need to be too concerned about this. The virus responsible for the common cold produces unpleasant symptoms but they do not carry with them the severe side effects that the influenza virus can.

The Spanish 'flu which wiped out more people at the end of the Great War than actually died as a result of this war, demonstrates the virulence of this enveloped virus.

There are many lipid coated viruses and bacteria and these include:

4

Lipid coated viruses
HIV Hepatitis C Measles Herpes simplex Herpes viridae Sarcoma Synctical virus Human lymphotropic virus Vesicular stomatitis virus Visna virus Cytomegalovirus Epstein-Barr virus Influenza Leukaemia virus Pneumonovirus

Lipid coated bacteria
Listeria monocytogenes Helicobacter pylori Streptococcus agalactiae Groups A, B. F & G streptococci Gram positive organisms Hemophilus influenza Staphylococcus aureus

---

4 The healing miracle of coconut oil, Bruce Fife N. D pg 61

Approximately 25% of the population are long term carriers of staphylococcus aureus (*S aureus*). It is found as in normal skin flora, in the lower reproductive tract of women and in the nostrils.

S aureus can produce a wide range of medical conditions including boils, cellulitis, pimples, abscesses, folliculitis and carbuncles, among others. However, it can also produce more severe infections which can be life threatening. These include:

- Meningitis
- Osteomyelitis
- Endocarditis
- Sepsis
- Toxic shock syndrome

S. aureus is one of the most common causes of hospital acquired infections and is generally the cause of wound infections following surgery. Thousands of deaths each year are *S. aureus* related with the elderly and those with compromise immune systems being mostly at risk.

S. aureus employs a number of defensive weapons which it uses to become resistant to many antibiotics. For example, staphylococcal resistance to penicillin is mediated by an enzyme, penicillinase. This cleaves part of the ring of the penicillin molecule which renders it effective. There are *B* lactam antibiotics such as flucloxacillan which are able to resist degradation by staphylococcal penicillinase.

Fortunately, coconut oil is effective against *S. aureus*.

The recommended dosage of coconut oil during illness is 4-8 tablespoonsful daily. This can be stirred into fruit juice to make It more palatable if this is preferred.

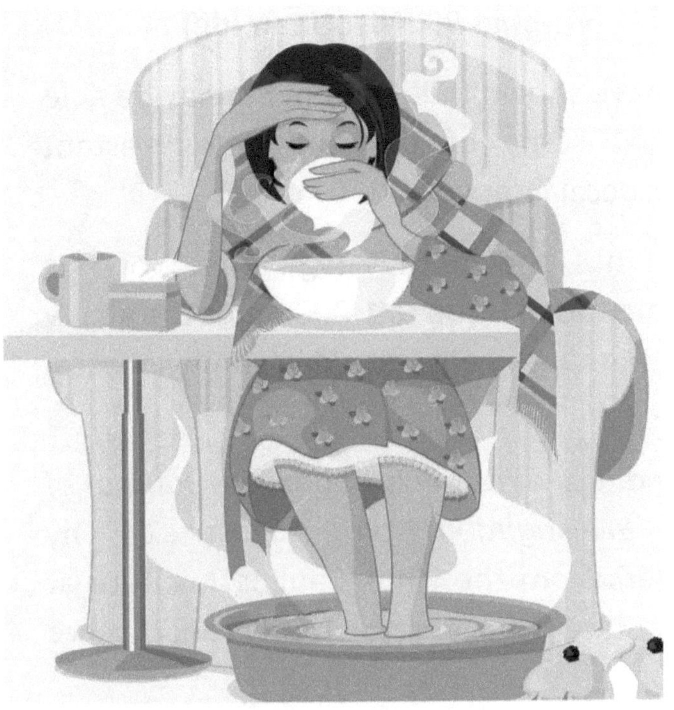

[5] Studies have shown that coconut oil is effective against the flu virus.

---

[5] https://pngtree.com/freepng/influenza-virus-infection_3097745.html

Vitamin B3 (Nicotinamide)

Studies have shown that vitamin B3 may be able to combat some of the antibiotic resistant staphylococcal infections.

Research has shown that high doses of this vitamin increased by up to 1,000 times the ability of the immune cells to kill staphylococcal bacteria.

These findings were published in the *Journal of Clinical Investigation* on August 27 by researchers from the Linus Pauling Institute at Oregan State University, UCLA and other institutions.

Vitamin B3 stimulates the innate immune system to provide a much more powerful response. In the case of vitamin B3, clinical doses of this increased the numbers and effectiveness of neutrophils. These white blood cells kill and eat harmful bacteria.

NEUTROPHIL

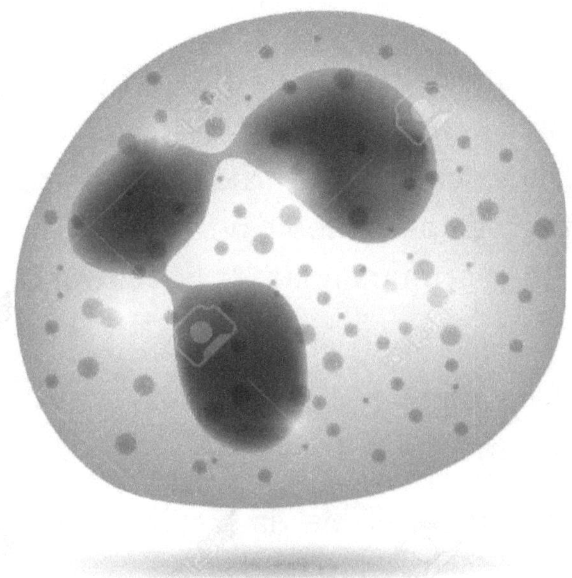

Further studies showed that clinical doses of vitamin B3 appeared to wipe out the staph infection in only a few hours.

It is not recommended that megadoses of this vitamin are taken routinely, without medical supervision, since high doses of vitamin B3 can damage the liver.

Given the potential negative side effects of mega doses of vitamin B3, a healthy balanced diet containing whole grains, mushrooms, peanuts, avocados and green peas should be the aim. This will provide the recommended daily allowance for vitamin B3 of

- 14mg for women
- 16mg for men.

Higher doses are available via prescription but are normally given to help lower cholesterol levels rather than to treat staph infections.

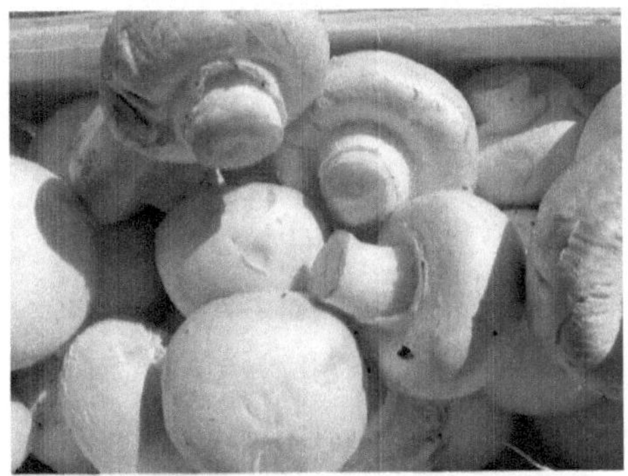

Mushrooms contain vitamin B3 and can help fight staphylococcus infections.

Mushrooms

It is perhaps fitting that we finished off the last section showing that mushrooms had the potential to kill off an enveloped bacterium. Mushrooms are thought to be one of the richest sources of natural antibiotics. It is thought that they evolved this way as they had to protect themselves from the often damp and dirty environment that they grow in.

  Many prescribed antibiotics are made from mushrooms. These include streptomycin and tetracycline. For example, Ganomycin, a powerful antibiotic is made from Reishi mushrooms. However, most mushrooms will have both antibacterial and antiviral properties although these will be of greater or lesser strength depending on the variety of mushroom.

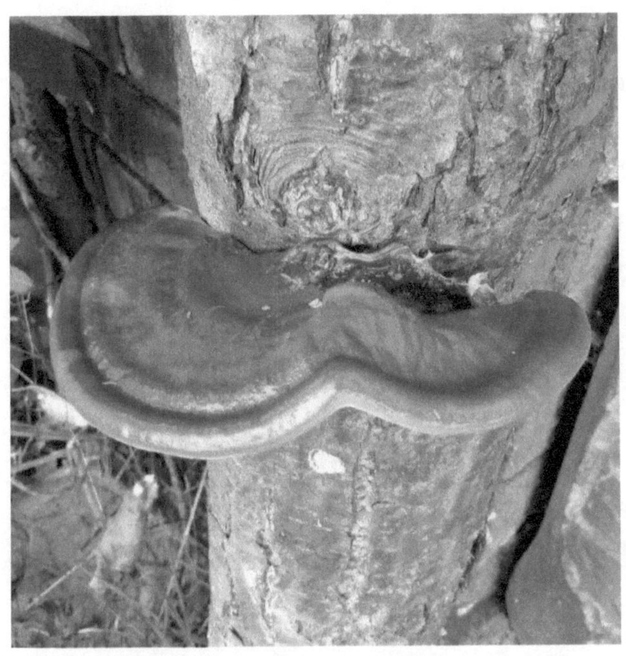

Ganomycin is made from Reishi mushrooms [6]

Ganomycin has also been found to be helpful in the treatment of metabolic resistance assisting in weight loss, insulin resistance, hypoglycaemia and hepatic steatosis.

Reishi mushroom is also capable of boosting your immune system and some forms of reishi are

---

[6] https://www.gourmetmushrooms.co.uk/shop/plug-spawn/reishi-mushroom-plug-spawn/

capable of altering inflammation pathways in white blood cells.

Research in cancer patients[7] has shown that some of the molecules found in the mushroom can increase the activity of a white blood cell which is part of the innate immune system. These are called Natural Killer cells (NK's).

Natural killer cells fight cancer and infections in the body. Other studies have shown that reishi can increase the number of lymphocytes in those with colorectal cancer.[8]

Lymphocytes are white cells that are vital to our immune system defences. There are three main types:

- T cells
- B cells
- Natural killer cells

---

[7] https://www.ncbi.nlm.nih.gov/pubmed/12916709
[8] https://www.ncbi.nlm.nih.gov/pubmed/16428086

Lymphocytes recognise invaders, produce antibodies and destroy any cells which could cause damage to us.

Reishi potentially has cancer fighting properties. One study showed that of over 4,000 breast cancer survivors, 59% of them consumed reishi mushrooms.

Other studies[9] did not find this link between reishi and anti-cancer effects although they did find an improved response to chemotherapy in those eating reishi.

It is thought that reishi should be used as an adjunctive therapy alongside traditional cancer treatment.

The five best mushrooms with antiviral and antibacterial efficacy were found to be:

.

---

[9] https://www.cancertherapyadvisor.com/fact-sheets/cancer-reishi-mushroom-fact-sheet/article/647081/2/

- Coliolus
- Reishi
- Shiitake
- Mitake
- Agarikon

Coliolus was found to be effective against both gram + and gram- bacteria. In S *aureus,* extracts from coliolus were found to elongate and cause malformation of their cells.   In Salmonella Enteriditis, colilolus was found to rupture the cells walls thus killing the bacterium.

Shiitake mushrooms were tested against 29 bacterial and fungal pathogens. It was found that there was extensive antimicrobial activity against 85% of these pathogens.

The antiviral and antibacterial effects came from such substances like:

- Oxalic acid
- Lentinan
- Centinanycins A and B

- Eritadenine (antiviral)

Agarikon is a huge fungus which hangs off trees

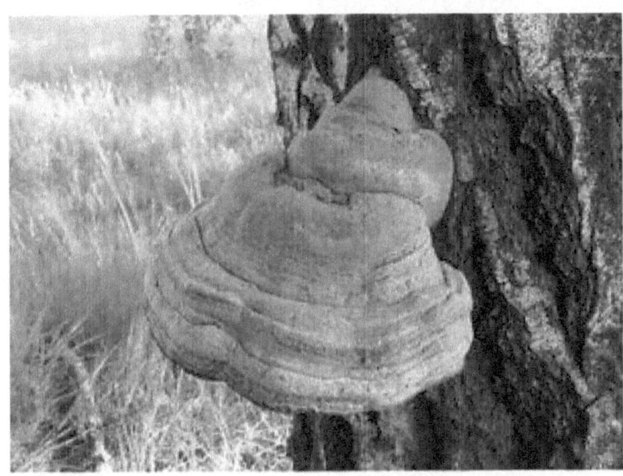

The fungus agarikon[10] has antiviral and antibacterial properties.

Studies show that agarikon showed efficacy against tuberculosis and that it also reduced inflammation as well as many other bacterial and viral infections. It shows strong activity against cowpox, swine and bird flu and the virus that causes herpes. Mycologist, Paul Stamets, noted

---

[10] https://www.ebay.com/itm/20-Fresh-AGARIKON-Fomitopsis-Mushroom-Plugs-Dowels-Spawn-Spores-Mycelium-/302264116278

that agarikon's effectiveness was better in some cases than conventional therapies.[11]

There are many powdered forms of mushroom on the market which can be bought through health food shops or online and which can be made into a tea, soup or added to a vegetable terrine, as wished. Be guided by the instructions on the packet and, if any side effects do occur then reduce the amount you are using. However, studies of reishi mushroom, in particular, show very few side effects, even when it has been used for an extended time.

---

[11] : https://phys.org/news/2014-10-mycologist-agarikon-possibility-counter-antibiotic.html#jCp

The healing power of garlic

Garlic has long been recognised as having antibacterial and antiviral properties but its ability to deal with infective agents goes well beyond this. Garlic is a broad spectrum antibiotic and its efficacy extends to antifungal

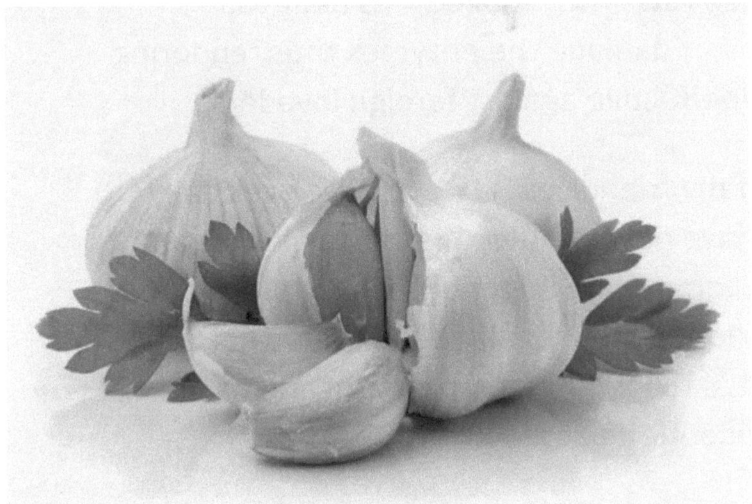

12

antiparasitic and antiprotozoan as well.

---

[12] http://humansarefree.com/2014/03/study-garlic-shrinks-tumors-up-to-74.html

Garlic is a bulb from the allium family and is well known for producing pungent breath when it has been eaten.

The active ingredient in garlic is allicin. It has to be eaten raw – not cooked – as heat will destroy or damage the enzymes thus rendering them ineffective against foreign invaders.

One of my friends eats two garlic cloves daily and I have never known him to fall ill with any of the community infections which appear to do their rounds on a regular basis. Garlic has the potential to lower blood pressure and has antioxidant effects, too.

Studies[13] have shown that garlic appears to have antibiotic activity whether it is taken internally or applied topically. Researchers found that the urine and blood serum of human subjects taking garlic had activity against fungi.

---

[13] Caporaso et al 1983

Many pharmaceutical antibiotics promote the development of resistant strains of bacteria. Garlic does not appear to produce these resistant strains of bacteria. Further, it may be effective against strains which have become resistant to pharmaceutical antibiotics.

Moore and Atkins (1977) tested garlic juice against a group of ten different bacteria and yeasts. They found that garlic was effective against all of them and they also found 'a complete absence of development of resistance.'

Garlic has also found to be effective against specific bacteria that are notorious for developing resistant strains such as staphylococcus, mycobacterium, salmonella and species of Proteus.

As antibiotics aren't effective against viruses, then they aren't effective against colds and flu. The viruses responsible for these are able to change shape so that they aren't recognised when they invade a body for more than one time. This is why it is possible to suffer repeated colds and flu. On the other hand, most people who get the common childhood illnesses like measles, mumps and chicken pox rarely get them more than once since these viruses a retain more stable structure. As such, if the virus tries to invade a second time, the body recognises it immediately and has defences already to deal with it – often before we are aware of any symptoms.

Garlic has been found to work against influenza, herpes, cowpox, vesicular stomach virus, (cold sores) and cytomegalovirus (a common secondary infection found in those with AIDS).

In an animal study,[14] researchers fed a garlic extract to some mice. They then introduced the flu virus into the nasal passages of the mice. The control group did not receive any diet of garlic.

---

[14] Adetumbi and Lau 1983

The mice fed the garlic were protected from the flu but the ones who didn't receive the garlic became sick.

The researchers hypothesised that the effects of garlic were partly due to its antiviral effects and partly due to stimulation of the immune system.

Garlic activates phagocytes which engulf invading pathogens, B cells and T cells. This is all the levels of the cellular immune system.

Garlic contains a substance known as diallyl trisulfide. This activates natural killer cells and macrophages. It also increases B-cell activity which subsequently increases the antibodies which attach themselves to pathogens and mark them for destruction.

Diallyl trisulfide treated macrophages were also found to be more active against cancer cells than macrophages not treated with diallyl-trisulphide. Not only was their number increased but their activity was too.[15] Studies with patients suffering from AIDS showed that two cloves a day given to ten patients for six weeks followed by four cloves of garlic for another six weeks revealed normal levels of natural killer cells when previously they had been low.

Opportunistic infections – infections which take advantage of a lowered immune system – such as sinusitis and genital herpes – improved. What is telling is that the patient with sinusitis[16] had not gained any relief from antibiotics.

Another study showed that a preparation of garlic powder given to elderly patients showed an increase in phagocytosis of the white blood cells ad also increased the number of lymphocytes.

---

[16] Abdullah 1989

Garlic and gums

Garlic has the potential to keep your gums healthy. A study published in the July 2005 *Archives of Oral Biology,* found that garlic inhibits disease causing bacteria in the mouth and has value in fighting periodontitis which is a serious gum disease. The supporting structures of the teeth become infected and inflamed. This will result in tooth loss.

Oral health is important because it has far reaching effects when it goes wrong. Pathogens from the mouth can get into the bloodstream, travel to the heart valve and damage it. Some studies[17] have also shown that mouth bacteria can be linked

---

[17]

https://www.nhs.uk/news/.../gum-disease-linked-increased-risk-alzheimers-disease/

to dementia. Gum disease sufferers were
70% more likely to get dementia.

Elderberries and pectin in apples.

We are very fortunate to have seven apple trees all of which are different varieties. We also have a pear tree, two plum trees, a damson and an elderberry tree among many of the plants we grow for their medicinal properties.

Our elderberry tree is a delight producing sprays of creamy sprays of flowers in summer and, in the autumn it is hung with tiny black gleaming powerhouses of antiviral goodness.

Studies[18] have shown that sambucol –its scientific name – was shown to be effective against 10 strains of influenza virus. Further sambucol reduced the duration of flu symptoms to 3-4 days

---

[18] Barak V[1], Halperin T, Kalickman I.

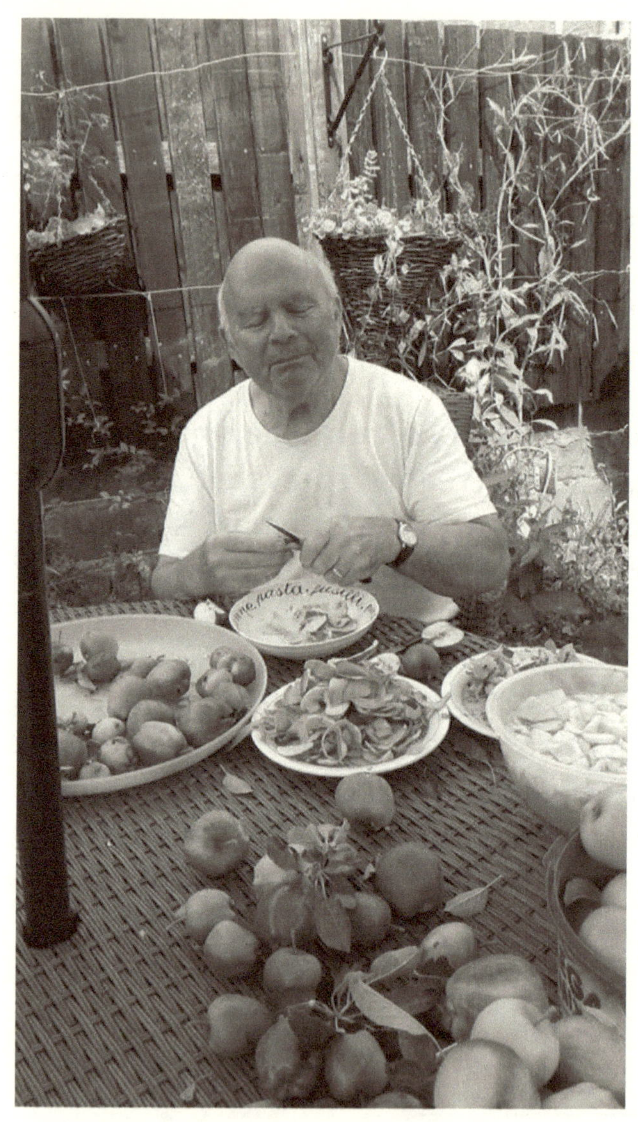

Michael peeling apples in our garden 2018

In the convalescent phase, serum taken showed a higher antibody level to influenza virus in the sambucol group than the control group.

A further study aimed to assess the effect of sambucol products on the healthy immune system – namely on cytokine production.

Cytokines are substances which are secreted by certain cells of the immune system and have an effect on other cells.

In this study, the production of inflammatory cytokines was tested using blood-derived monocytes from 12 healthy human donors.

Monocytes are a type of white blood cell which can change into macrophages which engulf pathogens. They are part of the adaptive immune system.

The results were that inflammatory cytokines were increased significantly demonstrating that not only did sambucol have antiviral properties but that it also had immune activating properties. Sambucol could also be beneficial for cancer or AIDS patients

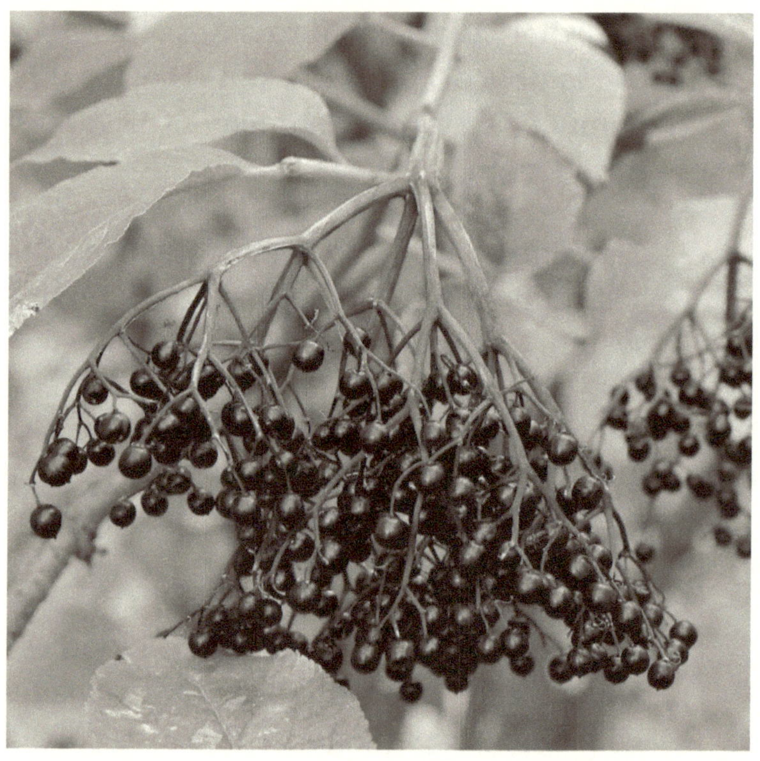

19

19 https://www.eatrightseattle.org/team/elderberry-syrup

Elderberries should never be eaten raw. They are a purgative. However, they are perfectly safe when cooked. I use them in pies with apples or make jam with them. Mostly I make elderberry syrup for the winter which comes in useful as soon as one of the winter infections makes its round. Elderberry syrup is also called elderberry rob. Here is one of my recipes which you can use to pour over pancakes as well as take as a medicine.

Ingredients
1 cup of black elderberries
4 cups of water
2 slices of fresh ginger
1 tsp of cinnamon powder
2-3 cloves
200ml of honey

Instructions

Pour water and all ingredients, apart from the honey, into a saucepan.

____

Simmer until the mixture has reduced by half.

Let cool and then strain. (this is the messy part). Mix the honey into the strained mixture and pour into a sterilised bottle or container.

This will store in the fridge but if I have made a large batch and don't intend to use it all within a month then I will freeze some of it until I need it.

Apples indirectly contribute to the health of the immune system through the pectin that they contain. Pectin is the substance in some fruits that helps jam set. Pectin is a type of fibre that acts as a prebiotic. This means it feeds the good bacteria in your gut.

A University of Illinois study found that soluble fibre, like pectin, reduces the inflammation associated with obesity related diseases and strengthens the immune system.

It appears that soluble fibre changes immune cells so that they go from being pro-inflammatory and angry to anti-inflammatory, healing cells which help us recover faster from infection. This occurred because soluble fibre caused increased production of an anti-inflammatory protein called inter-leukin-4.

I combine the power of apples and elderberries in jams and pies for the winter but, if I have a surplus of apples, as I have this year, then I add apples to soups and gravies.

Apple gives soup a delicious base. It somehow brings out and enhances all the other flavours that you have added to make your soup. It also helps thicken it. This is one of the beauties of adding it to gravy. It thickens the meat stock in a most delightful way. I don't just reserve it for pork. I find apple goes well with any meat and helps balance all the flavours. Even potato and apple mashed together make a delightful combination to go with a main meal.

Whenever I make a fruit pudding, the main ingredient is apple. It binds the other ingredients together in the way that egg does. It brings with it, its own sweetness so that less sugar is needed and of course it brings valuable soluble fibre to feed the gut bacteria.

Does insoluble fibre have the same impact on the immune system that soluble fibre does? In another study the impact of insoluble and soluble fibre was tested on mice. One group of mice was fed soluble fibre for six weeks and the other group was fed insoluble fibre. After this time, the mice were fed lipopolysaccharide. This is a substance that is found in bacterial cell walls.

It was found that the mice fed the soluble fibre did not get sick but the mice fed the insoluble fibre did.

It really does appear as though an apple a day keeps the doctor away.

Of course, besides apples there are a number of other fruits which contain pectin such as pears and an even greater number of foods containing soluble fibre.

From the beginning of October when our trees are ready to harvest we make jugs full of fresh apple juice and early Christmas puddings which are full of our apples. It is a time of the year that we look forward to very much. There is nothing like harvesting your own food (and medicine) so that we are ready for the winter and for the numerous infections which are rife at this time of year.

Curcumin

Curcumin is a natural component of the rhizome *Curcuma Longa* that is also known as turmeric. It is the popular yellow spice which is commonly used in Asian countries in cooking and for medicinal uses. In particular, it is used to treat inflammatory conditions. However, it has also been used to treat diabetes and various types of cancer. Curcumin has multiple effects

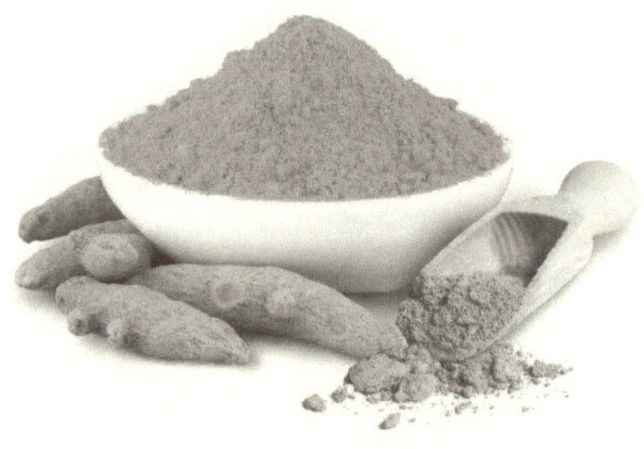

20

[20] https://www.indiamart.com/proddetail/pure-turmeric-powder-16143372297.html

and interacts with multiple targets that are involved in inflammation. These include:
- Interleukins
- Tumour necrosis factor

Interleukins (IL) are a group of naturally occurring proteins that bring about communication between cells. They regulate cell growth, differentiation and motility. They help stimulate immune responses such as inflammation, helping direct the battle against infection.

Tumour necrosis factor is another cell signalling protein which is involved in the acute inflammatory stage of an infection.

In vitro curcumin has been shown to possess in vitro antimicrobial action against a diversity of infectious agents including fungi and both Gram positive and Gram negative bacteria.

Studies[21] of curcumin showed that it stops *streptococcus mutans* sticking to human tooth surfaces and extra-cellular matrix protein.

---

[21] Song et al

Streptococcus mutans is responsible for tooth decay. *S.*mutans is a major pathogen of dental caries and is also known to be a causative agent of infective endocarditis.

Endocarditis is a rare and potentially fatal infection of the inner lining of the heart (the endocardium). It is most commonly caused by bacteria entering the blood and travelling to the heart.

In fact, poor dental health is a risk factor for many diseases which include Alzheimer's disease, yet it is overlooked as a major contributor to overall health.

Zinc

Zinc is a trace mineral which means it is only required in very small amounts. Nevertheless, zinc has some amazing abilities when it comes to destroying pathogens.[22] One of these is the bacterium, *Streptococcus mutans (S. mutans)* causing dental caries.

S. mutans learned how to survive in by producing large quantities of glucans and acid which exceeds the saliva's buffering capacity. It attaches itself to teeth and is more than able to survive in an acidic environment.

Zinc is also used as an antimicrobial. As such it has been added to toothpaste and mouth rinses. halitosis.

---

[22]

https://www.sciencedirect.com/science/article/pii/S101390521830 3237#b0100

Zinc – has great antiviral properties

A study[23] of Taiwanese patients with post herpetic neuralgia found that they were deficient in the mineral, zinc.

Zinc is a trace element. This means it is only required in very small amounts in our body. In spite of this, it has a number of important roles in the body.   Zinc is required to activate T lymphocytes (T cells). T cells are important because they:

- Help regulate immune responses

- Attack infected or cancerous cells

A study[22] found that the immune system was severely compromised when there was not enough available zinc and further, that zinc

<hr>

23

https://www.researchgate.net/publication/51033105_Nutrient_deficiencies_as_a_risk_factor_in_Taiwanese_patients_with_postherpetic_neuralgia deficient people were susceptible to a wide range of pathogens.

 The normal recommended dietary allowance of zinc is:

- 11mg for men
- 8mg for women

However, zinc can be taken in high doses (50mg) daily during a shingles outbreak. Zinc is able to inhibit the herpes zoster virus from replication.

Good sources of zinc include:

- Meat
- Shellfish
- Beans
- Eggs
- whole grains, seeds and nuts
- dairy

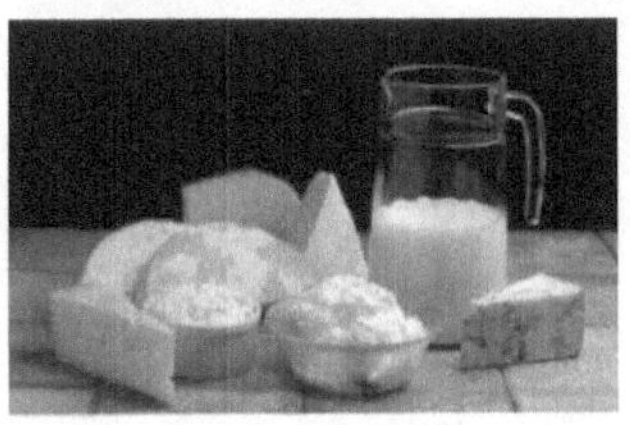

Is zinc effective for other diseases?

Zinc has a beneficial role to play in many other disease states. Studies have shown it to be effective in metabolic and chronic diseases that include: metabolic and chronic diseases such as diabetes, cancer, oesophageal cancer, breast cancer and neurodegenerative diseases.

Further evidence[24] exists for a link between zinc deficiency and a number of infectious diseases such as malaria, HIV, measles, pneumonia and tuberculosis.

Personal anecdote

My husband who is normally healthy, started suffering with sneezing, lethargy and cold symptoms. However, he maintained he was 'fine' so I didn't offer him any alternative medicine. By day four he felt, and looked, very poorly. His chest was rattling.

I, at this stage, started coming down with the same symptoms. I wasn't too happy about

---

[24] https://www.ncbi.nlm.nih.gov/pmc/articles/PMC5490603/

this so I took 50mg of zinc and gave my husband the same amount. My symptoms subsided overnight so that, by the morning I was back to normal and my husband was much improved.

 Zinc is one of those trace elements that should be kept in the medicine kit for times such as these. People who abstain from eating red meats as well as vegetarians and vegans are at a high risk of developing zinc deficiency as the amounts of zinc in plant based foods is insufficient to maintain adequate levels in the body. Further, a diet that contains mainly non-digestible plant ligands such as phytates, some dietary fibres and lignin inhibit the absorption of zinc.

Phytates are antioxidant compounds found in whole grains, legumes, nuts and seeds. They can bind to zinc (as well as other dietary minerals) and slow or inhibit their absorption

According to WHO[25], zinc deficiency is currently the fifth leading cause of mortality and morbidity in developing countries. It is estimated that it affects about one-third of the world's population.

---

[25] World Health Organisation . The World Health Report. World Health Organization; Geneva, Switzerland: 2002.

Lysine

Lysine is an essential amino acid which is well known for its anti-viral properties in respect to Herpes Simplex Virus (HSV). Lysine displays its antiviral effects by blocking the activity of arginine which promotes HSV replication.

Normally 1gm, given three times a day is the recommended therapeutic dose.

Rest

I have never yet come across a book on natural antimicrobials which actively encourages people to take time out to reflect and recover from the strains of modern life.

Not that many generations ago, people were encouraged to take to their beds if they had a fever or were unwell for any reason. Rest is restorative, it boosts your immune system to deal with the infection that is invading your body.

During sleep, your immune system synthesises infection fighting antibodies and cells occurs. These are reduced when enough rest is not taken.

According to Diwaker Balachandran, MD, Director of the Sleep Center at the University of Texas, MD Anderson Cancer Center in Houston there is experimental data to support the above.

In fact, sleep and the circadian system exert strong regulatory influence on immune functions. According to studies[26] of the normal sleep wake cycle naive T cells and pro-inflammatory cytokines peak during early nocturnal sleep.

Other immune system cells like natural killer cells and anti-inflammatory activity is at its best during daytime wakefulness.

When the immune system remembers past invaders this appears to have a particular association with the stage of slow wave sleep.

We shall come back to how to obtain a good night's rest shortly.

When we look at **moderate** exercise, we find that it, too, boosts the immune system. Moderate exercise results in a boost in the production of macrophages which are the cells which attack bacteria. The immune cells circulate through the body more quickly and are better able to kill bacteria and viruses.

---

[26] https://www.ncbi.nlm.nih.gov/pmc/articles/PMC3256323/

However, intense exercise can have the opposite effect. It appears to cause a temporary decrease in immune system function. This comes about because during intense physical exertion, the body produces certain hormones that temporarily lower immunity.

Cortisol and adrenalin, which are the stress hormones, temporarily lower immunity. Endurance athletes have an increased susceptibility to infection after marathon running or the intense training workouts that they are involved in.

Thus the importance of rest, relaxation, enough sleep and sunlight are just as true to our health as they were in our grandparent's day.

Our immune system has evolved to be able to cope with any diseases that come our way but most people do not consider their immune system as a vital contributor to their health. Why should they? After all they cannot see what a complex piece of mechanism it is. If they could they would treat it with more respect in the same way that a long saved for car is treated with reverence. It is maintained and cossetted and we expect it to serve us well and run for many years.

Our bodies are no different. If we treat them well then they will serve us well when it comes to the numerous infective agents that are waiting to invade our bodies. Further, nature has supplied numerous forms of adjunctive medicine which supports our innate and adaptive immune systems at times of illness. It is medicine for free once we have learned how to use it to our advantage.

Restorative Sleep

Sleep has a vital contribution to play in keeping the immune system running in tip top order. Two amino acids that help individuals gain good quality sleep are glycine and theanine.

Glycine is the smallest amino acid there is. It is non-essential which means that the body normally makes it from other substances and it is not essential to get it from food.

That is probably too simplistic a statement to make because all sorts of things can go wrong which hinders the synthesis of glycine. At the simplest level there may not be enough of the precursor nutrients to synthesise glycine.

Most of what we eat nowadays does not include the parts of an animal that contains the protein gelatin which has glycine as its main amino acids.

In fact, as our diets — and therefore our composition of amino acids changes, - then we can expect a new set of disease states to beset society.

Glycine is an inhibitory amino acid which means that it helps to calm things down. Anxiety lessens and pain is relieved. It restores sleep.

Glycine is found in many foods which have lost popularity nowadays. If supplementation is necessary, take 3g daily half an hour before retiring to bed or, at any time, in order to alleviate pain.

Table showing most popular foods containing glycine. [27]

Rank	Food Name
1	Gelatins, dry powder, unsweetened Glycine: 11374mg
2	Gelatin desserts, dry mix, reduced calorie, with aspartame, added phosphorus, potassium, sodium, vitamin C Glycine: 7983mg
3	Gelatin desserts, dry mix, reduced calorie, with aspartame, no added sodium Glycine: 7983mg
4	Snacks, pork skins, plain Glycine: 4382mg
5	Snacks, pork skins, barbecue-flavor Glycine: 4103mg
6	Pork, pickled pork hocks Glycine: 3910mg
7	Pork, fresh, variety meats and by-products, ears, frozen, cooked, simmered Glycine: 3787mg
8	Pork, fresh, variety meats and by-products, ears, frozen, raw Glycine: 3761mg
9	Beef, cured, luncheon meat, jellied Glycine: 3242mg
10	Chicken breast, oven-roasted, fat-free, sliced Glycine: 3124mg

---

[27] https://nutritiondata.self.com/foods-00009400000000000000.html

L-theanine

This is another amino acid which has calming effects and reduces anxiety. As such, it is very helpful in aiding sleep.

Theanine has very few sources and is only found in green or black tea. Perhaps the old habit of keeping cold tea and soaking dried fruit in it should be brought back such is its beneficial properties.

The feeling of calm and relaxation that we feel when we are drinking a cup of tea is entirely due to theanine's effects.

L-theanine has also been found to have some effects against *Staphylococcus aureus and Escherichia coli.*

Thank you for purchasing this book. Every time
a book is purchased, a donation is made to one
of the charities I am currently supporting.
These can be found on my author's website.
See below.

Other Health Related Books by the Author

- **The Reluctant Bowel**
- **A Weighty Issue**
- **Sleep, Perchance to Dream**
- **The Journey: EDS and chronic pain**
- **The MND diet: using nutrition to slow
  down the progress of neurodegeneration**
- **A Necessary Sorrow**
- **Taking another Road: Pain: its causes
  and what can be done about it.**
- **Pain associated with fibromyalgia,
  arthritis and soft tissue**

These can be found here on the author's page

https://www.amazon.co.uk/-/e/B07BPQZ5CD

You may also be interested in the semi-autobiographical trilogy of the authors life found in these three books

- The Prejudged
- Where the Blackbird Never Sings
- A Summer's Symphony

And the author's children's books

- Fanny and Victorian Jack
- Fanny and the Gamekeeper's Cottage